COMPLETE
COCONUT
GUIDE

OIL, MILK, AND WATER

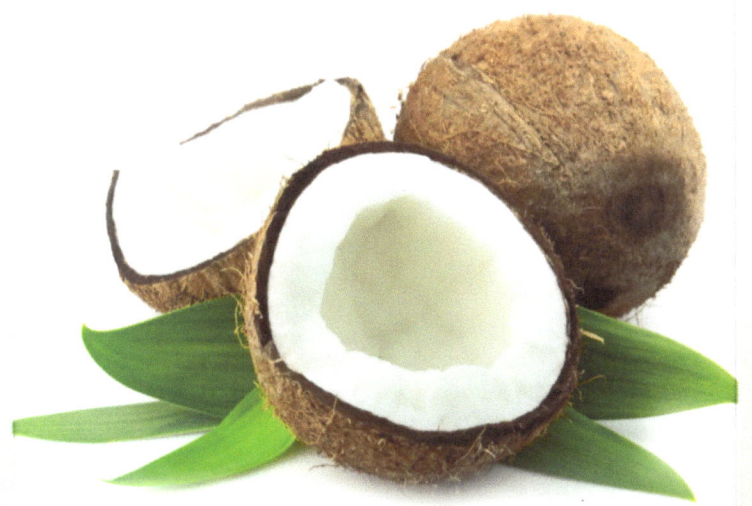

JESSICA SIMMONS

Coconut Oil, Coconut Milk and Coconut Water

By

Jessica Simmons

Disclaimer

Legal Notice: - The author and publisher of this book and the accompanying materials have used their best efforts in preparing the material. The author and publisher make no representation or warranties with respect to the accuracy, applicability, fitness or completeness of the contents of this book. The information contained in this book is strictly for educational purposes. Therefore, if you wish to apply ideas contained in this book, you are taking full responsibility for your actions.

The author and publisher disclaim any warranties (express or implied), merchantability, or fitness for any particular purpose. The author and publisher shall in no event be held liable to any party for any direct, indirect, punitive, special, incidental or other consequential damages arising directly or indirectly from any use of this material, which is provided "as is", and without warranties.

As always, the advice of a competent legal, tax, accounting or other professional should be sought. The author and publisher do not warrant the performance, effectiveness or applicability of any sites listed or linked to in this book. All links are for information purposes only and are not warranted for content, accuracy or any other implied or explicit purpose.

Table of Contents

Introduction

I want to thank you and congratulate you for downloading the book, **"Coconut Oil, Coconut Milk and Coconut Water"**.

This book contains proven steps and strategies on how to **bring the health benefits of the coconut-based products (oil, milk and water) into your life.**

But before helping you to incorporate all these products in your life and before providing you with recipes that will make it easy even for a beginner in the art of cooking to make healthy dishes and drinks out of these ingredients, you will first have to understand what coconut oil, milk and water are. You will first have to understand where they come from, how health experts look at them and how they can improve your life.

You should look at the eBook here at hand as a journey into discovering (and uncovering) the truths behind some of the world's most famous coconut products. In between health and myth, in between simply being delicious and being actually beneficial for your body, coconut oil, coconut milk and coconut water are some of the best things you can bring into your diet.

But, in order to reap all these benefits, you will have to know how to do it and why you are doing it. Hopefully, this book will provide you with all the answers to the questions you have related to these coconut foods and it will offer you with all the information you need in order to get healthier and in order to get a better quality of life as a result of having incorporated these foods into your diet.

Thanks again for downloading this book, I hope you enjoy it!

Coconut Oil and the Things You Should Know about It

Coconut oil has been out there for quite a while and it is probably one of the most debated healthy foods in the world of weight loss, cardiovascular disease control and medicine in general. The opinions always seem to be split when it comes to it, but outside of providing you with raw opinions that do not make much sense for an "outsider", you should first try to understand what coconut oil actually is and where it comes from – so that you can form an opinion for yourself and know how to screen fact-based opinions from myths and inaccurate information.

Coconut oil is a type of oil extracted from the kernel of the coconut fruit – that's something you probably know already. What you may not know however is that coconut oil can be extracted by using various methods and that this can make the entire difference in the properties the final product will have.

Basically, there are two main types of processing when it comes to coconut oil: wet processing and dry processing. When coconut oil is obtained through wet processing, the meat of the coconut fruit is taken out and dried (in sunlight, in fire, and so on). The product obtained this way is called "copra" and this will be mixed with various solvents in order to obtain the actual coconut oil. Other than coconut oil, a particular type of mash will be obtained as well – but that is not for human consumption and it is usually used in order to feed ruminants.

The wet method of extracting coconut oil is less used out there because it is not really economical. When coconut oil is extracted through the wet method, the meat of the fruit is not dried. In this case, the protein of the fruit produces an emulsion that is consisted out of water and oil. The oil used to be separated from the water through boiling, but this method is hardly used any longer because it produces a discolored type of oil. Instead, the emulsion is pre-treated using cold, heat, salts, enzymes, shock waves and various other methods. Then, the emulsion goes through a centrifuging machine which separates the actual oil from the water.

As you may suspect, this type of processing coconut oil is expensive because it normally requires a lot of investment to be made in machines that help producers separate the oil from the water. And even this way, it still does not yield as much final product as the dry processing does. As a matter of fact, it is believed that up to 15% less coconut oil is yielded by using the wet processing methods, even if you take into consideration the mash and the oil lost in the dry processing.

Normally, after extracting the coconut oil itself, producers also take it through a process that extends its shelf life. This can mean that they may add certain solvents that yield more coconut oil and extend the shelf life, that they remove particular types of fatty acids or that they use particular numbers they stick to through the processing. For instance, the right moisture content of the copra (below 6%), the right moisture content of the oil (0,2%), the right boiling temperature (266-305 Fahrenheit degrees) and adding salt and/or citric acid to the final product can add up time for the shelf life of the oil itself and it can make it less susceptible to rancidification.

Virgin coconut oil can be extracted both from using the dry method and from using the wet method. Even more, it is produced from fresh meat, from coconut milk and even from residue. For instance, some coconut oil producers take out the meat, dry it out and then use a screw press to extract the oil. Others choose to grate it, dry it until it reaches 10-12% and then use a manual press to extract the oil.

When the oil is produced from coconut milk, the meat is grated and mixed with water and then the oil is squeezed out. Also, some producers allow it to ferment for up to 48 hours and then remove the oil. In this case, the cream obtained is heated to remove any oil that may have remained. Last, but not least, some producers use a centrifuge to separate the oil from the water

At the other end of the whole coconut oil manufacturing industry lies the so-called "RBD oil". "RBD" stands for "refined, bleached and deodorized" and the oil obtained this way is taken through further processes that remove its coconut aroma and leave it completely tasteless and aroma-less. This oil is highly encountered out there both in home cooking and in cosmetics, industry and pharmaceutical products as well. During the RBD coconut oil processing, a hydraulic press is used and more than 60% of the total weight of the coconut itself yields into oil (which is a lot more than in the case of the virgin coconut oil).

Even more, RBD oil is sometimes subject to hydrogenation as well, which basically makes unsaturated fats become more saturated. Some of them become trans fatty acids and therefore, the health quality of the oil is lowered considerably.

Health organizations, as well as organizations dealing with maintaining the standards of the food products out there have been equally interested in making sure that people know what they buy (and even more, that they know what they put in their mouths). Thus, the Asian and Pacific Coconut Community (whose members, by the way, produce over 90% of the world's total amount of coconut oil) have struggled to define what virgin coconut oil actually is. Eventually, they got to the conclusion that coconut oil should be labeled as "virgin" only when the product is obtained from fresh meat which has been processed without altering the oil itself (thus, hydrogenation and other methods to increase shelf life and melting points are not accepted under the "virgin coconut oil" label).

As you may already suspect, the kind of coconut oil you should incorporate in your diet is the virgin type. Yet, if you want to know how to tell if a particular type of oil is of high quality, you should not simply trust what the label says, but you should also know how to "test" it yourself. Here are the main criteria for detecting high quality virgin coconut oil:

1. It should be really white when solid and it should be really clear when melted. Usually, if there is a yellow shade in it, then it means that it will be of a lower quality. Even more than that, stay away from any type of coconut oil that shows other colors because it will most likely be contaminated either with mold or smoke residue. Both of these contaminators are signs that the coconut oil has been obtained through some sort of dry processing (which consequently lowers the oil's quality)

2. High quality virgin coconut oil actually smells and tastes like coconut, but it will be a mild aroma, not a very strong one. If you "bump" into coconut oil that smells and tastes like nothing, it is most likely obtained through RBD-specific methods.

3. Even more, if it tastes or smells like anything but coconut, stay away from it as well because it has been contaminated. Likewise, coconut oil that has a very poignant coconut flavor or aroma is not a good option either.

4. It is approximately OK if the coconut oil has a slightly roasted coconut flavor/aroma, but it will still mean that some sort of heating process was used (and that the oil was not obtained through wet processing).

5. Last, but definitely not least, be wary of any coconut oil that is too inexpensive. As shown throughout this first chapter, when a lot of coconut oil is yielded, "unorthodox" means were used and the oil is anything but virgin. The real virgin coconut oil is yielded from large amounts of coconut and its processing is not a very fast one, which means that producers will need to add up on the price at least a bit so that they can make profit. Bottom line is that you do get what you pay for when it comes to coconut oil. The cheapest one will be most likely RBD-processed (or, in any way, not 100% virgin), while the slightly more expensive ones stand a much better chance at being actually virgin and unaltered.

Coconut Milk and Coconut Water: the Things You Should Know about Them

Coconut milk is a liquid obtained out of coconut meat. In most of the Western countries, it is bought in cans and people do not obtain it through homemade processes, but in those places of the world where coconut grows naturally, people actually make their own coconut milk the same way as people in the West make their own cheese, sour cream and other products.

The process through which coconut milk is obtained is fairly easier to understand than that through which coconut oil is. Basically, this "milk" can be obtained through simply grating and squeezing the coconut through a cheesecloth. When this particular method is done, the milk obtained will be thick. However, thinner coconut milk can also be obtained if hot water is mixed into the thick coconut milk. Thick milk is mostly used in desserts and in making thick sauces for various dishes, while thinner milk is used in a wide variety of other recipes.

Canned coconut milk is the most commonly encountered type of coconut milk in the Western countries out there. Very frequently, milk separates in the can and this results in a creamy paste that floats right on top of the can. Some of the people use that as coconut cream, but a lot of people believe that this is a sign of spoilage. However, you should know that coconut milk that is perfectly evened out usually contains various types of emulsifiers.

To avoid canned coconut milk that is not 100% pure, you can either buy virgin coconut milk and simply shake it before using (because this will bring the whole can at the same consistency level) or you can make coconut milk at home. The process is quite simple and inexpensive and other than water and dried coconut flakes, you will not need much else in terms of tools and equipment (or at least not much else you don't already have around your house)

Basically, you need to combine 8 ounces unsweetened coconut flakes and 4 cups of nearly boiling water into a blender. Allow the flakes to soften up a bit by letting everything rest for a few minutes. Then, blend the mixture on high until you obtain a paste (you will still have some flakes here and there). Take a nut milk bag (you can find these for sale online and in natural products stores as well) and place it over a bowl. Take the coconut mixture and place it inside. Squeeze well. Everything that comes out is your coconut milk. Store it in mason jars or other glass-made storing items and use it as you please.

Coconut water is another liquid product obtained from coconut and the process of obtaining it is even easier to that through which coconut milk is obtained. In fact, in most of the cases there is no process at all, as the coconut itself contains this water. While ripe coconuts also contain water, the most frequently used fruits for this purpose are green coconuts that have not yet reached maturity.

Coconut water is very popular in tropical areas where the fruit grows naturally. You can find it on streets, you can drink it right from the fruits (and there are people who make a little "show" out of serving you coconut water right from the coconut itself) and you can also find it in tetra packs, in cans or in bottles as well (which is how most of the people in the Western countries obtain this great "water", since coconut does not grow naturally outside of the tropical climate area of the Globe).

All the 3 coconut-based foods presented in the first two chapters of this eBook can have tremendous health benefits and now that you understand how they are obtained (and how you can see if a product is of a high quality and it is unaltered), you can make the difference between the various types of products available on the market as well.

Following, this book will present you with health-related information on coconut oil, coconut milk and coconut water and it will try to dispel some of the myths and misconceptions that have been going around the topic of these 3 types of ingredients/juices obtained from coconut.

Hopefully, the pieces of information presented next will help you determine for yourself if you will want to incorporate coconut oil, milk and water into your diet or not. After reading what this eBook has to say, you will most likely be aware of these products' advantages and disadvantages and you will be able to make the best decision for your body, for your mind and for your general state of well-being as well.

As you will see, if you want to achieve success in reaping the benefits of these products you will have to keep in mind one simple word: "balance". By being fully aware of what these products actually do with your body, you will also know how to incorporate them into your diet correctly.

Coconut Oil: Healthy or Not So Much?

Coconut oil has been present on the Western food market for a long time now, but over the course of the years it has also been debated much among health specialists.

At first, there was not much concern regarding coconut oil – but then again, health specialists started to be really concerned with the effects fats have on cardiovascular health a bit later on. When research started showing that not all fat is "created alike", health specialists started to put coconut oil in the category of the so-called "bad fats".

For a very long time, coconut oil has been isolated in that group until rather recently when a new wave of attention got coconut oil. The last one decade or so has been very prolific in revealing new information about health and people generally started to become more health conscious than they used to be. Coconut oil was among the foods taken "out of the dark" and shown to the world as a not-so-bad-food-as-people-thought-it-was. In fact, the later research showed that coconut oil may actually possess health-enriching qualities other types of fats did not have.

However, if you want to truly understand the truth behind coconut oil and how healthy it is (or isn't - and when that happens), you should first understand what the deal with fats actually is. Again, this will help you judge things for yourself instead of simply accepting what the latest "health guru" has to say.

Fats: Between the Good, the Bad and the Evil

For a very long time there, dieticians advised against eating fatty products. Anything that contained fats was banned and there were multiple reasons for which nutritionists did this. For example, they believed that any kind of fat will bring damage to one's cardiovascular system. Even more (and this stands valid nowadays as well), one gram of fat contains 9 calories, which is much more than what one gram of protein or one gram of carbohydrates that contains 4 calories. Thus, it was a logical assumption to say that avoiding eating fats will lower the total caloric intake and it will avoid becoming overweight or obese.

That is true, indeed. Excess calories do make people put on weight.

But the truth revealed by the later research showed that fats are not as bad as people thought they were. As a matter of fact, they are extremely important for the good functioning of your entire body:

- You need fats to provide your body with the necessary energy it needs in order to function. On a normal burning rate, the body will first burn the calories taken from carbs and only then it will start burning the fats. That means that your body will have to have some sort of fuel to get itself going after the carbs have been burned up.

- You need fats in order to maintain your health and your skin fresh and beautiful –and this is not true just for cosmetic products, but also for your nutrition. Fats help with the assimilation of vitamins A, D, E and K – all of them essential for the good health of your hair and skin.

- You need fat to keep your body warm. Fat acts like a "blanket" that protects your body from getting cold and this is one of the reasons for which anorexic people usually feel colder than normal-weighing people.

- You need the so-called "essential fats" for the good functioning of your brain, if you want to control inflammation and if you want to control blood clotting. These essential fats (linoleic acid and linolenic acid) are called "essential" for a reason: your body needs them, but it cannot produce them itself (thus, you will need foods that contain them).

All in all, living a completely fat-free life and taking out all the fatty foods from your diet is not a healthy choice (and it cannot be sustainable on the long-term no matter how you look at it). Eating less fat does not necessarily mean that there will be less fat on your body. For instance, if you eat very few fats, but indulge in a lot of carbs, you will get nowhere because carbs are transformed into sugars when they reach the blood stream and any kind of sugar that is not properly "burnt" will store itself as fat on your body. Even more, this kind of diet can lead you to develop very serious health conditions – such as diabetes for example.

Going back to fats though, you now know that you should not be avoiding them completely from your diet. Yet, all the health professionals out there say that a diet that is high in fats will lead to serious health conditions as well: blood and circulation conditions (such as clogged arteries), heart diseases, stroke, diabetes, digestive issues and many, many other health-related issues.

What is there to do then and who should you believe? Should you stop eating fats or should you continue eating them? What kind of approach is the best one to actually maintain your body healthy and strong or as long as possible?

The absolute truth about fats can be found somewhere in the middle of the above-mentioned directions. That is, you should eat fats. But even more than that, you should eat the *right* types of fats – the ones that get you going and the ones that are good for your body. At the same time, you should be avoiding the *wrong* types of fats – the ones that clog your arteries, rise the cholesterol levels (the "bad" cholesterol levels, to be more precise) and the ones that are normally found in most of the foods that have been labeled as "unhealthy" for at least a couple of decades now (such as fast food products, many of the packaged meals, fried meals and so on).

So, which are the fats you should eat and which are those you shouldn't?

Put simply, there are 3 types of fats out there, found in various types of foods:

1. Saturated fats are among the worst ones and they are responsible for rising bad cholesterol levels (LDL cholesterol, to be more precise). High levels of this cholesterol cause heart attacks, cancer and many other diseases and medical conditions as well. Basically, this type of cholesterol builds up in your arteries as a wax-like substance that clogs arteries and makes blood circulation more and more difficult.

   Most often, saturated fats are found in animal products (such as butter, cheese, ice cream and meats with a high percentage of fat, for example). There are some "tropical oils" that contain high levels of saturated fats as well. Palm oil is one of them and another one among these tropical oils is the subject of the ebook itself – coconut oil.

   You should limit your saturated fats intake to a maximum of 10% per day if you want to stay healthy and to avoid having your body build up excess LDL cholesterol.

2. Trans fatty acids are also very bad for your body. Trans fats are usually obtained when the vegetable oil is hydrogenated; a process that hardens it up and then melts it so that its shelf life is extended. What trans fats do is not only pushing the LDL cholesterol levels up, but also lowering the HDL cholesterol as well (this is actually the "good" type of cholesterol your body needs in order to function properly). Margarine and hard butter are both known to contain a lot of trans fats, but so is coconut oil that has been hydrogenated as well.

3. Last, but not least, unsaturated fats are those that lower the LDL cholesterol. There are 2 main types of unsaturated fats: mono-unsaturated and polyunsaturated. In most of the cases, mono-unsaturated fats are found in oils such as olive oil and canola oil and polyunsaturated fats are found in sunflower oil, soy oil, corn oil and other oils as well. As a rule of thumb, you should know that most of the oils that are liquid at room temperature contain unsaturated fats (either mono or poly).

As you can see, the story about fats and which ones are healthy and which ones are not is actually more complex than some dieticians in the past believed. You may feel that you know everything you need to know about coconut oil already, but the truth is that with this oil, things get even more complicated.

Yes, coconut oil contains saturated fats - and this is one of the main reasons for which health professionals have been banning it into the group of foods that should be avoided as much as possible. Like with all saturated fats, coconut oil can make the LDL cholesterol go up, but what you don't know already is that it can make the HDL cholesterol go up as well, thus making the damage on the body be significantly lower. This makes coconut oil a better alternative to butter, shortening and other types of saturated fats that you may now include in your diet.

One tablespoon of coconut oil contains about the same amount of calories and fats as one tablespoon of olive oil. However, the coconut oil contains about 88% saturated fats, while olive oil only contains about 15% saturated fats.

The debate on coconut oil goes much further than this as well and it is important that you understand all the facets of consuming coconut oil before you incorporate it in your diet with a certain amount of regularity.

For example, it was mentioned above that coconut oil can contain hydrogenated fats (trans-fats). However, you should keep in mind the fact that this is only true for coconut oil that has been hydrogenated and altered, not for virgin coconut oil. With virgin coconut oil, things are completely different.

Since everyone seems to be claiming that coconut oil is extremely healthy then, which are the benefits that are brought as argument to sustain this idea?

1. As already mentioned, it is a good alternative to other types of saturated fats. Instead of butter, coconut oil can make for a better food and many have replaced their saturated fat intake with it.

2. It is a great alternative for those people who are, for example, dairy-intolerant. Many people find that their bodies cannot process dairy-based products properly and they find themselves in the situation where they have to give up on these foods completely. Coconut oil can make for a butter substitute and it can replace butter and other milk-based products in cooking various kinds of dishes (from main courses to deserts).

3. It is a great ingredient for those on diets such as Paleo or for vegetarians. Both of these diets remove dairy products from one's nutrition, but coconut oil (and, as you will later on see, other coconut products as well) can make for a great replacement.

4. Coconut oil may be high in saturated fats, but they are of the medium-chain triglyceride type. These MCTs (medium-chain triglycerides) are metabolized differently by the body and they can help one lose weight because they provide the body with energy that is more long-lasting than that in other types of saturated fats out there.

   This is one of the main reasons for which people have been advising for using coconut oil in many weight loss programs out there and why many others have seen a lot of good results too. Even more, the fact that coconut oil is rich in MCTs means that the body will burn more calories in one day (up to approximately 120 calories), which can lead to weight loss over the long term.

Furthermore, research has been done and some claim that coconut oil can help people not only lose weight, but lose it from the abdominal area, which is one of the most dangerous areas your body can store fat in because it can be a sign that you are prone to develop heart-related conditions and diabetes as well.

5. Coconut oil contains lauric acid – which is, as mentioned before, one of the two main types of essential oils the human body needs. This means that coconut oil has anti-inflammatory and anti-microbial effects and that it can be used successfully in treating acne, as well as in disinfecting various things. It may seem like a paradox that something so oily can treat acne, but it is true indeed.

6. Even more, it has been shown in some studies that virgin coconut oil can help with reducing certain inflammatory diseases, such as arthritis. Although there is not very much evidence, this is definitely something worth looking into.

7. Also, it has been claimed that coconut oil can help patients suffering from Alzheimer's. This can be true and although there is no precise data to reveal a certain pattern in this, there have been people whose Alzheimer's got improved once they started to increase the coconut oil intake.

8. If you look at the nations where coconut oil is highly consumed, you will find out that they are actually very healthy and that even if they do have the highest saturated fats intake, they don't develop as much heart diseases as people in the Western countries. Tokelauans are one such example, but there are many others as well.

9. Coconut oil has also been shown to fight hunger. It has been shown that people who eat coconut oil are more likely to feel like eating less than normally and even more, that people who integrate coconut oil into their breakfasts are likely to reduce the number of calories they eat at lunch as well.

10. Coconut oil is one of the power foods used in the ketogenic diet. This diet has been out there for almost 100 years and ever since it was "developed" it attracted everyone's attention. A ketogenic diet can be used in managing children who suffer from epilepsy, but some of the people claim it can also help with weight loss as well. Basically, this diet will focus on eating larger amounts of "good" fats and on eating smaller amounts of carbohydrates (often times, very small amounts of them, actually).

11. Coconut oil has been used outside of kitchen for quite a long time as well. Here are some of its uses that may (or may not) be surprising for you:

    a. Coconut oil can be used as a moisturizer. Simply whipping coconut oil and applying it on your body can "feed" your skin with a lot of good things that will make it shine more and that will make it be younger.

b. Coconut oil can be used as a sunscreen as well. Same as with the moisturizer, you can simply apply it on your skin to get a more beautiful tan and to protect your skin from malevolent sunlight.

c. Coconut oil can lie at the basis of other cosmetic products as well (including, but not limited to eyeliner, lipstick, lip gloss and so on)

d. Coconut oil can be successfully used for polishing furniture. Simply using it as it is will bring back the shine in your furniture.

e. Coconut oil can be applied on the hair as a mask to regenerate it and to make it shinier.

f. Coconut oil can be used to lubricate guitar strings.

g. Coconut oil can be used when you want to remove chewing gum from clothes, shoes and even from the hair.

h. Coconut oil can be used as a part of various masks that fight acne (again, this may seem surprising, given the fact that coconut oil is fat, but it actually works).

i. Coconut oil can be used to remove head lice.

j. It can be used to treat eczemas and other irritations.

k. It can be used as a local disinfectant on smaller wounds.

l. Coconut oil can prevent your nose from running bloody and dry when the dry season kicks in.

m. Coconut oil can be used to make homemade, healthy and chemical-free deodorant.

n. Coconut oil can be used to whiten teeth and it can be part of a homemade tooth paste recipe as well.

o. Oil pulling is an Ayurvedic practice that involves swishing coconut oil into the mouth and spitting it out. This is said to help with migraines, whiten teeth and also to help with detoxifying the body in general.

p. "kalpa vriksha" is the Sanskrit word used to describe the coconut and it roughly translates as "the fruit which gives everything necessary to life". The naming is quite revealing for the many properties coconut in general can have and for the many uses coconut oil as a product made from coconut can have as well.

As you can see, coconut oil can seem almost miraculous both when it comes to the number of uses it can have and when it comes to the efficiency with which it can help you in all of these uses.

As a recap, what does coconut oil contain that makes it stand out from the "crowd" of the many other types of oils and foods?

1. It is high in saturated fat, but not just any kind of saturated fat, but in MCTs, which are actually good for weight loss.

2. It increases LDL cholesterol, but it also increases HDL cholesterol, which definitely puts less strain on your heart.

3. It contains essential oils such as linoleic acid which is good for the functioning of your brain.

4. It contains vitamin E, essential for the health of the skin, of the eyes and a means of reducing the risks of developing Alzheimer's, rheumatoid arthritis, male infertility and many other conditions.

5. It contains vitamin K, which protects the bones and helps with blood clotting as well.

6. As a fat, it helps absorbing vitamins A, D, E and K absorb easier into the body even when they come from other sources.

To answer the question of the title, yes, coconut oil is healthy. BUT (there is a "but") you should not take any kind of coconut oil as being healthy. The refined, bleached and deodorized versions, as well as those coconut oils that have been hydrogenated will not be good for your health. The virgin coconut oil, however, will be healthy for you. Sadly, in this case you do get what you pay for because coconut oil that is virgin and non-refined is usually more expensive. However, considering the fact that your health is actually at stake, it is a small price to pay.

Even more than that, you should keep in mind that nothing in the world that is consumed in excess will ever be healthy. Take the banal apples, for example. Everybody knows them and everybody knows the saying "an apple a day keeps the doctor away". Indeed, apples are extremely healthy for your body because they contain a myriad of vitamins, fiber and anti-oxidants as well. However, eating too many apples can also mean that you will be getting a lot of fructose in your body, which is essentially a type of glucose and which should not be found in large amounts in a healthy body.

The same thing goes for coconut oil as well. Consume it in moderation and wisely, in recipes that are actually worth it and you will reap its benefits. Consume it excessively and obsessively and you may see the darker side of the properties this oil has.

In the end, it is all about the quality of the oil you use and about the amount you use as well, which can stand valid for most of the foods out there as well. Balance is the key to integrating coconut oil successfully in your diet and you should keep that in mind with every single food you eat.

Coconut Milk: Health Benefits

Coconut milk is quite a commonly encountered product in most of the supermarkets out there and, the same as with coconut oil it has been much debated in the entire health industry out there. The claims for coconut milk and its potential health risks go mainly the same as with coconut oil as well and, as you will discover throughout the following chapter, the health benefits go the same as well.

Basically, health professionals are concerned that coconut milk may contain too much saturated fat, even as compared to fat cow milk. However, the same explanation as in the case of coconut oil works here as well. The saturated fat contained by coconut milk is rich in medium-chain triglycerides, which basically means that it will be a non-typical type of saturated fat: the kind that actually makes people lose weight.

Even more, the other health benefits of coconut oil go for coconut milk as well. It can reduce the risk and lower the development of Alzheimer's (as well as other cognitive diseases such as Parkinson's, for example), it can help the skin and the hair look much better, it can help with the better functioning of the brain, it can help with increasing both LDL and HDL cholesterol, and the list goes on and on. Even more, coconut milk is known to help the immune system function better as well, particularly due to the high content of the lauric acid, which is very good for this purpose.

Other than healthy saturated fats, coconut milk also contains vitamin C, E, B1, B3, B5 and B6, as well as a series of minerals that are needed for the good functioning of the human body (iron, selenium, calcium, magnesium and so on).

Also, you should know that you can opt for low-fat coconut milk. You can either find it canned and labeled as such, or you can make it at home by following the recipe presented in the first chapter of this ebook and by adding more warm water to make it thinner.

Coconut milk can be found in cans, but the healthiest choice is fresh coconut milk. However, since this is not widely accessible in the Western world, you may want to opt for making it yourself. Do bear in mind that bought fresh coconut milk should be used as soon as possible and that homemade coconut milk should not be stored for more than 3-4 days in the refrigerator, in air-tight container. Canned coconut milk can be stored in your cupboard at room temperatures for months in a row, but do bear in mind that you should read the label and see if it contains sugar (which is the kind of coconut milk to be avoided) and to see when it expires.

What is coconut milk used for, though?

Everything cow milk is used for – and more. Coconut milk is encountered in many Asian and Pacific cuisines, including Thai, Vietnamese, Chinese, Burmese, Filipino, Indian, Malaysian, Brazilian, Polynesian and in the Pacific Isles.

It is used in a wide variety of dishes, ranging from slow cookers to curries and from baked goods to the classic American pancakes. It can give food a particular type of flavor, but normally, high quality coconut milk should not be very poignant in the coconut taste and aroma it has (the same way as high quality coconut oil is not this way either).

Also, coconut milk is used in many drinks as well. Some of them are alcoholic, some of them are not. In South China and in other Asian and Pacific counties, coconut milk is mixed with cow's milk and sold as such, as a refreshing drink. In other countries, it is mixed with coconut cream to create Pina Colada, as well as with other ingredients to create various types of cocktails.

Healthy smoothies very frequently contain coconut milk as well. These smoothies can be very easily made at home and they contain coconut milk for its taste, for its health benefits and for the fact that it can replace dairy successfully. Basically, there is an almost limitless number of combinations that can be made with coconut milk, vegetables and fruits so that you obtain a delicious and extremely healthy smoothie (which can be a great breakfast, a dinner, an energizer before working out or a snack in between your main meals).

Furthermore, when it is allowed to rest uncovered the refrigerator, coconut milk will usually split and there will be a layer on top of the container that will resemble cream. Many people use that as a whipped cream replacement since it can be whipped and then added to deserts the same way as normal whipped cream.

Even more than that, coconut milk is a great alternative for people who are lactose-intolerant. Lactose is one of the enzymes the human body finds quite difficult to process and many people out there have bodies that do not allow them to eat lactose because it comes with adverse effects. Bloating, cramps, gurgling sounds in the lower belly, gas, diarrhea, nausea and many other symptoms are associated with this condition.

Since lactose-intolerant people avoid eating any kind of dairy product, milk is not part of their diet. Thus, coconut milk, being of a vegetal origin, can replace cow milk successfully in their diet. Although it does not have the very same properties (it does not contain as much calcium as cow milk does), coconut milk has the same texture and the same sweet-like taste as cow milk does and it can make for an especially great replacement especially in baked goods and cakes.

In addition to people who are lactose-intolerant, there are many other people who follow dairy-free diets as well (for various purposes). For instance, the famous Paleo diet involves eating only foods people in the Paleolithic era used to eat and it is based on the idea that grains and many other products (dairy products included) are not good for the human body simply because it has not yet gotten used to digesting them properly. Thus, processed foods and anything that may contain gluten or lactose is banished from the diet. This leads to people having to search for various replacements and coconut milk (as well as coconut oil and even a so-called "coconut flour") is used very much in the recipes labeled as "Paleo".

Vegans also eat a lot of coconut-based products and this is so because they will not eat anything that is produced by an animal (eggs, milk, dairy, meat, fish and so on). Thus, if you open a vegan (or vegetarian) labeled cookbook, you are very likely to find a lot of recipes that contain coconut milk and other coconut-based byproducts (oil, flour, cream).

Is coconut milk healthy?

Yes, most certainly so. But, same as in the case of most of the foods out there and same as in the case of coconut oil, you have to know how to consume it in moderation and to know how to choose it the right way. Generally speaking, health professionals advise for incorporating about 1-3 portions of coconut milk every week, but do bear in mind that they speak about the thinner versions and about the unsweetened versions. Also, avoid coconut milk cans that have suspiciously long shelf life and that contain preservatives. All in all, reading the label can definitely make for a great difference so do it because it will cost nothing at all!

Coconut Water: Is It Good for Your Body?

Many people out there take coconut water as being one and the same with coconut milk, but the difference between them is very big and you should be aware of this.

Basically, coconut water is normally obtained out of green coconuts, although the ripe ones contain coconut water as well. This "water" is basically the juice that can be found inside the coconut kernel and it can be simply drunk as such. In the countries where coconut grows naturally, the people selling it frequently drill a hole in the fruit and serve the water from it directly. However, do bear in mind that coconut fruits that have fallen out of the tree are not normally used because they are susceptible to being rotten or damaged by animals or insects.

Also, you should definitely know the fact that coconuts have to be at least 5 months old if you want the water in them to be proper for drinking. Anything younger than that will not have the same health benefits (described later on) and not even the same taste as the good coconut water (as it will taste bitter instead of sweet).

One green coconut can contain anything between approximately 7 ounces of coconut water and 33 ounces of it. However, ripe coconuts contain much less coconut water because their water has been absorbed into the meat (and there will be more meat on them as compared with green coconuts). The amount of coconut water that can be found in a green coconut depends on various factors, including the particular type of coconut and its size.

In addition to being drunk as such, coconut water can also be used to make coconut vinegar as well and it can be incorporated in numerous recipes, from banal pancakes to delicious smoothies to energize and nourish the body as well.

One interesting thing you may want to know about coconut water is that it is normally sterile. In case the fruit has not been altered, the water in it should be free of any bacteria or contaminators. This has led people to using it as an intravenous replacement to a saline solution. The story goes that this happened in the World War II in the case of the British and Japanese soldiers because the doctors did not have any saline solution supplies at hand. However, this practice is not used any longer because it has been discovered that coconut water contains a lot of potassium and calcium, which is why it may become dangerous when it reaches the bloodstream.

And here's another interesting fact: coconut water is traditionally used in India for senicide (the suicide committed by the elderly members of the family). According to this tradition, elderly people are given an oil bath in the morning and then they drink coconut water in excess, until their kidneys fail and until the fever fits become very high. Within 1 or 2 days, most of these people die.

However, that does not make coconut water evil or dangerous for one's health and life. In fact, even water can kill if consumed in excess. In fact, coconut water is extremely healthy for one's body and it shows properties different than coconut oil and coconut milk, especially in the way it can help the human body get healthier and fitter. If you want to find out more about this, then here are some of the most well-known health benefits of coconut water:

1. It is a great refreshing drink. As long as it does not have any added sugars, coconut water can replace any soda – both from the point of view of the taste and from the point of view of the satisfaction it will give you. Of course, water is best, but coconut water can really replenish your body with enough nutritional factors to get yourself going through a hot day of summer.

2. As a matter of fact, coconut water is so rich in various types of minerals that it has been dubbed as "nature's sports drink" and the truth is that it can really energize your body when you have a session of working out at the gym in mind. Coconut water contains fifteen more potassium than man-made (non-natural) sports drinks, which is very good considering your body will need a lot of potassium to be replenished with after a workout session because it will lose this mineral through sweat. Also, your body will need magnesium since this mineral makes your muscles function well.

   However, what coconut water will contain in smaller quantities than normal sports drinks is sodium, which is also lost through sweat. If you are planning on a medium-intensity workout session though, coconut water can be more than enough (and it can be a much healthier alternative to sweetened and full-of-colorants-and-chemicals sports drinks).

3. Coconut water has been administered for diarrhea for quite a long time now. The reason it works so well when this medical condition arises is related to the fact that diarrhea tends to dehydrate the body severely and coconut water is known to be rich in minerals and nutrients that replenish one's body's mineral "stocks".

4. If you thought other fruits and/or vegetables are rich in minerals, then you should really know the fact that coconut water contains more calcium, manganese, magnesium, iron and zinc than many of the other fruits out there (including more of this minerals than oranges show – and everyone knows that oranges are packed with minerals and vitamins).

5. Same as coconut milk, coconut water is very rich in B-mineral complexes which are absolutely essential for the human body but which are not naturally produced by it.

6. If you have access to fresh coconut water, you should know the fact that it also contains Vitamin C, which is very much known to be a great improver of the immune system and a great anti-oxidant as well.

7. Furthermore, it has been shown that coconut water contains cytokinins, which are known to be anti-aging and anti-carcinogenic ingredients as well.

8. Also, coconut water can help boost the metabolism and help with digestion due to its bioactive enzymes (such as acid phosphatase, dehydrogenase, peroxidase and RNA-polymerases as well).

9. Coconut water has been hailed to be a great helper for those who aim at losing weight. Because it contains low amounts of fats (surprisingly, considering that the other coconut-based products actually do contain quite a lot of fats), it can be consumed in larger quantities. Even more, it has the quality of making one feel full as well.

10. Like all the other coconut-based products (milk, oil, cream and so on), coconut water can help you get a better skin as well. If you consume it, your skin will look more moisturized and it will not have as much excess oil as normally. If you apply the coconut water topically, you can treat acne since this "water" is a very good anti-inflammatory "potion" as well.

11. Although it is definitely not advised to ever drink as much as to get yourself with a hangover the next morning, the truth is that this happens to some of the people out there. Coconut oil can be a natural remedy because it replaces the essential electrolytes the body loses through drinking alcohol (because these beverages dehydrate the body instead of hydrating it and the hangover is nothing but the series of symptoms that arise from this).

12. Coconut water can also be efficient in reducing blood pressure. Sometimes, this medical condition appears as a result of a certain imbalance of the electrolytes in blood. Since coconut oil is very rich in electrolytes, it can help lowering the blood pressure.

13. Coconut water is compatible with the human blood and, as mentioned in the beginning of the chapter, can be administered intravenously as a hydration solution. Yet, this is not so much advisable any longer due to the high contents of calcium and potassium that are found in this water.

14. Pregnant women find coconut water to be beneficial for them as well, especially because it helps with digestion, it helps with heart burn symptoms and it fights off constipation as well.

15. Also, it is believed that coconut water can be considered to be a highly efficient diuretic and that it is good for the kidneys (as long as it is not

consumed in excess, the way in which it has been described in the beginning of the chapter).

Of course, these are just some of the most important health benefits that come with consuming coconut water, but there may be many more "unchartered" ones out there as well. Even without all these amazing benefits, coconut water can still make for a delicious and refreshing drink that will always be much, much healthier than any kind of bought beverage.

Delicious Coconut Recipes

As you have seen throughout this ebook, coconut is extremely healthy in all its variations: coconut oil, coconut milk and coconut water and coconut water. Of course, it should be consumed in moderation, but that is valid for anything else out there (even for the common apple).

Also, you should know how to consume it correctly, in recipes that are healthy, nutritious and delicious as well. For instance, eating deep fried dishes and using coconut oil will not make you reap any of its benefits. Instead, incorporating coconut oil in healthy dishes will bring you with a lot of health benefits you will definitely want to reap.

To help you and to give you an idea of just how great dishes with coconut oil, coconut milk and coconut water can be, this ebook has put together a few delicious and healthy recipes that are very easy to make and that will definitely be to the taste of every single member in your family (even the capricious little ones).

1. Coconut Curry Recipe

As it was already mentioned, coconut oil has been present in the Indian cuisine for a long time. Naturally, there will be a lot of curry recipes to contain coconut oil and coconut milk as well. Here is one of the simplest and most delicious ones:

Ingredients:

2 tablespoons red curry paste

2 tablespoons virgin coconut oil

2 cloves garlic, minced

1 onion, chopped

4 cups coconut milk

2 chicken breasts, sliced (thin)

1 stalk lemongrass, bruised and cut

3-5 Kafir lime leaves

Some basil

Directions:

In a large skillet, bring the coconut oil to the melting point and add the curry paste in it. Sauté it for about 2 minutes and then add the onions and the garlic. Sauté until they are cooked (onion should be slightly translucent and garlic should emanate a specific aroma).

Add all the other ingredients (outside of the basil), reduce the heat, cover and allow everything to simmer for about 30 minutes until the chicken is cooked through.

Serve on a bed of rice (Jasmine or Basmati) and top with some basil for garnish.

2. Coconut Steak

Steak may not be the healthiest dish out there, but you are allowed to indulge in it every once in a while as long as you use meat that is as lean as possible. This particular recipe works with any kind of steak and it will be maddeningly delicious as well.

Ingredients:

2 cups water

1 cup coconut water vinegar

1 cup apple cider vinegar

4 cloves

2 bay leaves

2 onions, chopped

Salt and pepper

1 steak

1 tablespoon coconut oil

Directions:

Outside of the coconut oil and the steak, bring all the other ingredients into a pot and boil them. Pour over the steak while still hot and allow it to marinate overnight in the refrigerator.

Take the steak out and cook it in coconut oil.

This particular recipe works fabulously with mango chutney, but it can be eaten in any way you eat your steak normally.

3. Coconut Veggie Scrambled Eggs

Veggies are undoubtedly healthy and incorporating some eggs into your weekly menu is also a healthy choice. If you top everything with coconut oil, you'll get a real treat for your mind, for your soul and for your body as well – a treat for a perfect late Saturday morning.

Ingredients:

1 tablespoon virgin coconut oil

2 tablespoons zucchini, chopped finely

1 tablespoon onion, minced

2 cherry tomatoes, quartered

1-2 eggs

1 tablespoon coconut milk

Sea salt

Black pepper

Directions:

Bring the onions and the zucchinis into a sauce pan in which you have heated the coconut oil. Sauté them until they are tender.

Add the cherry tomatoes and sauté them as well.

Meanwhile, beat the egg with the milk and season it to taste.

Pour the egg mixture over the vegetables and scramble.

Serve hot and enjoy!

4. Vegetarian Coconut Mushroom Soup

Mushrooms are very good for your health if you know how to eat them right and soups are generally a very healthy choice. Consuming soups as often as possible will lower your daily calorie intake (because most of them are really low in calories) and will help your digestions as well. This recipe here will be very easy to make (especially since it uses a slow cooker) and it will be very tasty as well, so everyone in your family will love it.

Ingredients:

1 cup boiling water

1 pounds fresh mushrooms of your choice, trimmed and sliced

2 onions chopped (finely)

4 cloves garlic, minced

½ teaspoon dried thyme leaves

1 teaspoon sea salt

½ teaspoon black peppercorns, cracked

1 bay leaf

4 cups organic vegetable broth

1 cup coconut milk

4 tablespoons virgin coconut oil

Directions:

Start by soaking the mushrooms in the boiling water for about 30 minutes. Sieve them well and make sure there is no water left in them by patting them with paper towels. Reserve the mushroom water used. Chop them finely. Split in two parts and reserve one of the parts for later on in the process of making the soup.

Add one tablespoon coconut oil to a pan and bring the mushrooms there. Cook over medium heat until they lose all the water. Transfer them to a slow cooker

Use the same pan and add the remaining coconut oil to it. Sauté the onions there. Add the reserved mushrooms, the garlic, the thyme, the peppercorns and the salt and cook everything for about 1 minute. Transfer the mixture to the slow cooker

Add the bay leaf, the broth, the mushroom water and the coconut milk to the slow cooker as well. Stir very well so that everything is combined perfectly.

Cook on low for about 6-8 hours or on high for about 3-4 hours. Discard the bay leaf and serve hot.

5. Coconut Granola Bars

Granola bars work very well with yogurt and kefir and they definitely make for a healthy and tasty breakfast as well. If you want to make your own granola bars and incorporate some coconut in them, then this recipe will work very well.

Ingredients:

15 cups rolled oats

2 cups walnuts, chopped

4-5 cups unsweetened coconut flakes

3 tablespoons cinnamon

10 ounces brown rice syrup

2 cups melted coconut oil + 1 teaspoon or more for the cookie sheet.

Directions:

The first step you have to make is to preheat your oven at 350 degrees and to oil a cookie sheet using the coconut oil reserved for this.

Bring all the dry ingredients together. Then, slowly add in the coconut oil and the rice syrup.

Pour half of this mixture unto the cookie sheet and cook for 5 minutes.

Take it out, stir and cook for another 5-7 minutes.

Do the same with the other half of the mixture as well.

6. Banana Coconut Muffins

Alright, muffins are not a very good dietary choice – but they are good for your soul. Even more, the muffins here contain no dairy and no gluten, which makes them suitable for many people. For a special breakfast, they are definitely worth giving a try.

Ingredients:

½ cup walnuts, chopped

1 cup bananas, mashed

½ cup raw honey

½ cup coconut flour

1/3 cup melted coconut oil

3 eggs

½ teaspoon sea salt

½ teaspoon baking soda

Directions:

Start by preheating the oven to 350 degrees.

Put cupcake liners into your muffin tins. Also, you can grease with coconut oil (extra oil from the recipe ingredient list) and you can dust with coconut flour (also, not from the recipe ingredients list)

Mix mashed bananas (they should be creamy) with honey.

Add the coconut flour, the coconut oil, the eggs and the salt. Use a hand mixer and mix everything thoroughly for about 1 minute.

Allow the mixture to sit for about 2 minutes

Add the baking soda and the walnuts to the mixture. Stir quickly until the baking soda is incorporated.

Fill your cupcake forms and bake them until they are browned. You can use a toothpick to insert and see if it comes to clean to tell if the muffins are actually done.

7. Green Coconut Smoothie

If you want a refreshing, energy-packed and incredibly healthy drink for your breakfast, then this coconut smoothie here will be everything your body and your heart may desire.

Ingredients:

1 cup water or ½ cup water and ½ cup ice

4 cups pineapple

½ cup coconut milk

1 cup spinach

Directions:

Star by blending ice and the water for a few seconds.

Add in the spinach for a few seconds more.

Add the remaining ingredients and blend until it has a smooth texture. This may take up to 10 minutes in the case of the slowest blender out there.

Conclusion

Thank you again for downloading this book!

I hope this book was able to help you to understand coconut oil, coconut milk and coconut water better, as well as the health benefits that come with them (and how they can actually be beneficial).

The next step is to purchase high quality coconut oil, coconut milk and water and start incorporating it into your diet in a balanced and well-thought out way.

Finally, if you enjoyed this book, please take the time to share your thoughts and post a review on Amazon. It'd be greatly appreciated!